AF367718

Ketogenic Diet Meal Prep

Weight Loss Cookbook with Breakfast, Lunch, and Dinner Recipes

By: Sebastian Beach

© Copyright 2016 by Sebastian Beach- All rights reserved.

This document is geared towards providing exact and reliable information in regards to the topic and issue covered. The publication is sold with the idea that the publisher is not required to render accounting, officially permitted, or otherwise, qualified services. If advice is necessary, legal or professional, a practiced individual in the profession should be ordered.

- From a Declaration of Principles which was accepted and approved equally by a Committee of the American Bar Association and a Committee of Publishers and Associations.

In no way is it legal to reproduce, duplicate, or transmit any part of this document in either electronic means or in printed format. Recording of this publication is strictly prohibited and any storage of this document is not allowed unless with written permission from the publisher. All rights reserved.

The information provided herein is stated to be truthful and consistent, in that any liability, in terms of inattention or otherwise, by any usage or abuse of any policies, processes, or directions contained within is the solitary and utter responsibility of the recipient reader. Under no circumstances will any legal responsibility or blame be held against the publisher for any reparation, damages, or monetary loss due to the information herein, either directly or indirectly.

Respective authors own all copyrights not held by the publisher.

The information herein is offered for informational purposes solely, and is universal as so. The presentation of the information is without contract or any type of guarantee assurance.

The trademarks that are used are without any consent, and the publication of the trademark is without permission or backing by the trademark owner. All trademarks and brands within this book are for clarifying purposes only and are the owned by the owners themselves, not affiliated with this document.

Table of Contents

Introduction

This book contains proven steps and strategies on how to go on the keto diet and prepare delicious and nutritious keto meals.

Learn how the keto diet works and how you can get started on it. Find out which foods are keto-approved and how to create meal plans based on these guidelines. Most importantly, learn how to prepare a variety of keto breakfast, lunch, and dinner meals that are chock full of the nutrients and energy that your body needs.

This book was written for anyone who wants to lose weight, manage type 2 diabetes, and reduce his or her risk of developing cancer and other debilitating diseases. It is also for anyone who is curious about the keto diet and would like to understand it as well as give it a try.

Get started on the keto diet now and transform your body into a high energy fat-burning machine!

Thanks again for downloading this book. I hope you enjoy it!

Chapter 1 – How to Get Started: Keto versus Normal Diets

The ketogenic diet, often called *keto* for short, is described as high in fat and low in carbohydrates. It was originally designed to help those with epilepsy cope with their medical condition, but studies later on revealed that the diet can also help reduce the risk of the development of type 2 diabetes, cancer, and Alzheimer's disease. This is because the keto diet can significantly reduce insulin and blood sugar levels.

To be on the keto diet, you need to significantly reduce your intake of carbohydrates and instead get your daily source of energy from fat. After approximately two weeks of being consistently on the keto diet, your body will eventually get into the state of *ketosis*. During this state, the body will start transforming the fat stores in the liver into ketones which will be then be used as its main source of energy.

The keto diet is completely unique from other diets because it is concentrated on the consumption of high amounts of fat. Normal diets, on the other hand, focus on deprivation of not just carbohydrates but also fat. This means you do not have to "starve" your body. In other words, you can still enjoy delicious and nutritious meals throughout the day.

The Types of Keto Diets

There are four main types of keto diets, each of which is designed to address specific needs. These are: the Standard Ketogenic Diet (SKD), the High-Protein Ketogenic Diet, the Cyclical Ketogenic Diet (CKD), and the Targeted Ketogenic Diet (TKD).

- **Standard Ketogenic Diet** – this type of keto diet is characterized as extremely low in carbohydrates (approximately 5 percent), regular in protein (approximately 20 percent), and high in fat (approximately 75 percent). This ratio is to be followed in every meal with no exceptions.

- **High-Protein Ketogenic Diet** – while this type of keto diet is almost the same as the SKD; the big difference is in the increased protein intake. Hence, the ratio for this diet should be 5 percent carbs, 35 percent protein, and 60 percent fat.

- **Cyclical Ketogenic Diet** – this type of keto diet is a cyclic system between a primarily keto diet with brief high carb feeding intervals. The common practice would be five days on the keto diet followed by two days on the high carb diet before going right back to the keto diet.

- **Targeted Ketogenic Diet** – this is a special type of keto diet that is meant for those who work out regularly, especially among athletes. Specifically, it involves adding some carbohydrates before each intensive workout.

It is imperative that you consult your doctor before following the keto diet because the state of ketosis does have detrimental effects on certain people, especially those who are at risk of heart attacks, stroke, atherosclerosis, and other cardiovascular diseases.

It is equally important to work with a licensed fitness expert if you plan to follow the keto diet with a sound workout program. For those who wish to follow it for weight loss, then it is best to consult a dietitian in order to determine your daily caloric and nutritional needs and to match them with the appropriate meal plans.

Common Myths Regarding the Keto Diet
It is only natural to be skeptical of a diet, especially one that is controversial due to the fact that it highly encourages fat consumption. To help debunk the myths and clear the fog, below is a list of the true answers to the common concerns with regard to the keto diet:

Myth #1: You can't build muscles on the keto diet.

This one is false because you definitely can build muscles with the keto diet. However, this can only be effectively achieved with the Cyclical or Targeted Ketogenic Diet types than with the Standard or High-Protein types.

Myth #2: You will frequently feel fatigued when you are following the keto diet regularly.

Partly false, because if this occurs then your body may not be properly transforming your fat stores into ketones that should serve as your main source of energy. If you experience fatigue even after two weeks into the keto diet, then you should do your best to eliminate carb intake and consult your physician regarding supplements such as MCT oil.

Myth #3: I can no longer eat carbs for the rest of my life when I'm on the keto diet.

This one is false, especially if you are exercising regularly (see the Cyclical or Targeted Ketogenic Diets). However, it is imperative that you completely eliminate carbs within the first 60 to 90 days into the keto diet. After that, you may eat small amounts of healthy sources of complex carbohydrates during special events.

Myth #4: I will experience muscle mass loss with the keto diet.

Partially true. However, take note that *any* type of diet that eliminates a macro nutrient (in this case, carbohydrates) will trigger muscle mass loss. If your goal is to increase muscle mass, then you should choose the Cyclical or Targeted Keto diets.

Myth #5: If I follow the keto diet, I will suffer from mild halitosis (or bad breath).

This is a normal side effect of ketosis, but it is a minor setback that can easily be addressed if you drink mint tea or lemon water regularly, or if you chew sugar-free gum.

Myth #6: The keto diet will cause my pee to smell fruity.

This is another side effect of ketosis and should not be something of concern, unless your urine is of an unusual color.

Myth #7: Ketosis is life-threatening and not worth the health benefits of the keto diet.

False. Ketosis is often confused with ketoacidosis, which is a condition that takes place when a person with diabetes does not do anything to control his or her condition. Ketosis, on the other hand, is natural. Nevertheless, consult your doctor before starting the keto diet for safety reasons.

How to Get Started on the Keto Diet

Now that you have a general idea of what the keto diet is all about and what to expect from it, you can now put your knowledge into action. Here are the steps on how to get started:

Step 1: Consult a Health Professional to determine whether or not you can start the keto diet.

Step 2: Determine which type of keto diet is ideal for you based on your health and fitness goals.

Step 3: Design a meal plan and collect recipes that are sustainable for you depending on your lifestyle and personal preferences.

Step 4: Clean out your kitchen to get rid of any foods that you should avoid while on the keto diet.

Step 5: Create a grocery list of the food items you need for your meal plan.

Step 6: Research online on where to purchase the best quality and most affordable food items in your grocery list.

Step 7: Shop in bulk for your food items.

Step 8: Prepare your keto meals.

Keep in mind that you will need to make a conscious effort in sticking to your keto diet. Ideally, you should incorporate a regular workout regimen as well. This will require loads of self-discipline, especially if you have gotten so used to the conventional, carb-filled diet.

Be determined and constantly motivated, and eventually the keto diet will become second nature to you. Soon enough, you are well on your way to becoming strong, lean and full of energy.

Chapter 2 – The Ketogenic Diet Food List

The Ketogenic diet is all about fresh, natural ingredients. You should choose only the best produce that your budget can afford so that you can get the most amount of nutrients from each serving.

That being said, here is the comprehensive list of foods that you should stock up on when following the keto diet:

Healthy fats and oil
Fat is the primary source of energy in the keto diet, therefore most of your daily caloric needs should be from fats. Healthy fats should be in the form of Omega-3 fatty acids, such as from wild-caught salmon, tuna, and other fatty fish. If fish is not a good option for you, then you should consider taking fish oil supplements. Omega-6 fatty acids are also important in the keto diet. You can get them from eggs, nuts, and poultry. Make sure to choose the organic, whole foods kind.

Monounsaturated fats or the "good" fats take center-stage here. You can get them from olive oil, avocados and nuts. Choose the certified high quality "cold pressed" oils to ensure that you are regularly feeding your body with the right kind of fat.

Saturated fat is not considered a bad thing in the keto diet just as long as they come from organic sources, such as grass-fed butter and organic meat.

In a nutshell, you should stock up on the following healthy sources of fats and oil:

- Monounsaturated fats such as olives or olive oil, avocadoes and avocado oil, and macadamia nuts or macadamia oil.

- Polyunsaturated omega-3 sources, such as fatty fish and sea food.

- Saturated fat such as coconut oil and organic red meat (beef tallow, chicken fat, and non-hydrogenated lard).

Avoid at all costs anything that is hydrogenated and partially hydrogenated as these contain trans fats, or the most life-threatening fats that are linked to coronary heart disease.

Reduce consumption of inflammatory Omega-6 sources, particularly in the form of sunflower oil and corn oil.

Organic Meats

Protein is important in the human diet and you therefore should consume some, but it should be eaten in moderation in the keto diet. You should get your protein from certified organic sources that are locally produced and abundantly available in your area. This will ensure that you are feeding your body right and nourishing your muscles appropriately for optimum muscle mass gain.

By choosing local, organic and unprocessed meats, you are also significantly reducing your risk of consuming unhealthy hormones, additives, and other toxic substances that are linked to cancer and other debilitating diseases.

Here is a list of the different sources of protein to consider in the keto diet:

- Wild-caught fatty fish such as cod, flounder, mackerel, salmon, halibut, tuna, snapper, trout. If possible, purchase the fish fresh from the fisherman's wharf. Then, chop them into appropriate serving sizes, salt them, and pack them in your freezer to extend their shelf life for up to several weeks. Make sure to rinse off the sodium before cooking.

- Wild-caught shellfish such as crab, oysters, mussels, squid, scallops, and lobster.

These should also be bought fresh from the fisherman's wharf and stored in the same way as fish.

- Free-range (organic) eggs.

It is much better to find a local source such as a nearby farmer's market or a local farmer to obtain your eggs instead of buying the pre-packaged ones at the supermarket.

- Poultry such as duck, chicken, turkey, quail, and pheasant.

Opt for free-range fowls from ethical local farmers instead of from industrially produced ones as the former have higher quality protein and fat.

- Meat such as beef, lamb, goat, pork and wild game. Choose grass-fed, pastured organic meat whenever possible because these contain significantly higher levels of fatty acid that your body will need.

Dairy Products

Full fat, organic milk products are ideal in the keto diet. This includes cheeses and creams. Some of the most commonly used milk products are:

- Buttermilk
- Cheddar cheese
- Colby cheese

- Cream cheese
- Feta cheese
- Monterey Jack cheese
- Mozzarella cheese
- Swiss cheese
- Heavy cream
- Sour cream
- Whole milk

Vegetables

Your main source of nutrients in the keto diet should come from leafy greens and other vegetables. Ideally, these should be locally produced, organic, and in-season to ensure freshness, optimum nutritional value, and of course, cheaper prices.

Here is a list of vegetables that are low in carbohydrates. If any of these are too expensive or unavailable in your area, search online or call your local nutrition center to identify the best alternatives.

- Kale
- Spinach
- Bok choy
- Chard
- Chives
- Endive
- Radicchio
- Kohlrabi
- Bamboo shoots

- Lettuce
- Cabbage
- Asparagus
- Broccoli
- Carrots
- Cauliflower
- Celery
- Cucumber
- Garlic
- Green beans
- Mushrooms
- Onion
- Bell pepper
- Shallots
- Snow peas
- Spinach
- Squash (such as acorn, butternut, and spaghetti)

Nuts and Seeds

Plenty of nuts and seeds are used in the keto diet and the generally preferred way to prepare them is through roasting. Take note that peanuts are legumes and should be consumed in small amounts in the keto diet.

Here is a list of the nuts and seeds commonly consumed when you are on the keto diet:

- Almonds
- Cashews
- Chestnuts

- Chia seeds
- Coconuts
- Flaxseeds
- Hazelnuts
- Macadamia nuts
- Pecans
- Pistachios
- Pumpkin seeds
- Sesame seeds
- Walnuts

Beverages and Sweetener

It is important to drink lots of water each day, especially when you are on the keto diet. This is because the diet is naturally diuretic, which means you will need to visit the toilet regularly. If you are not careful, you could also end up getting dehydrated. Keep a container full of fresh drinking water with you at all times and stay hydrated.

Aside from water, you can also enjoy black coffee and herbal tea. Avoid everything else except for keto-approved smoothies. If you have to sweeten your drinks or food, then use liquid stevia.

Chapter 3 – Create Your Own Keto Meal Plan

Your personalized keto meal plan should be more than just a list of the foods that you are supposed to eat each day. Rather, it also serves as your guide so that you will not stray from or cheat on your diet. Preparing meal plans ahead of time will help you save a lot of time, money and effort put into preparing your own keto meals at home.

That being said, here are the steps on how you can create your own keto meal plan:

Step 1: Determine how many calories your body needs in a day.

There are five main factors that determine how many calories your body needs each day in order to function properly, and these are your height, weight, age, sex, and activity level. It is important to take note of these before going online and finding an online "daily caloric needs" calculator.

For example, if you are a 27 year old woman who weighs 128 pounds and is 5 feet 1 inch tall and does no exercise at all, then the online calculator will reveal that you need about 1500 calories a day to maintain your current weight. If your goal is to lose weight, then you need to consume no more than 1000 to 1200 calories per day.

If you would rather calculate manually, then follow this formula to determine your basic metabolic rate:

For men: 66.5 + (13.75 x weight in kilograms) + (5.003 x height in centimeters) – (6.755 x age in years)

For women: 655.1 + (4.35 x weight in pounds) + (4.7 x height in inches) – (4.7 x age in years)

For instance, if you are a 28 year old man who weighs 77 kilograms and is 177.8 centimeters tall, then you should calculate your BMR this way:

66.5 + (13.75 x 77) + (5.003 x 177.8) – (6.755 x 28) = 1825.64

This means you need to consume 1825.64 calories per day to maintain your weight, less 200 or so calories to lose weight and the other way around to gain weight.

Take note that you need to burn 3500 calories to lose one pound and vice versa.

Step 2: Identify the times when you can have meals.

Ideally, you should eat three regular meals and three small meals per day, especially when you are on the keto diet. To be more specific, your everyday meal plan should consist of:

- 1 Breakfast
- 1 Morning Snack

- 1 Lunch
- 1 Afternoon Snack
- 1 Dinner
- 1 Evening Snack

Each meal should be about 3 to 4 hours apart so that you will avoid "feeling" hungry, which in turn will make you more likely to succumb to your food cravings. It is important to stick to this healthy eating habit and you can make it easier for yourself by setting timers to remind you that it is time to eat.

For example, you can set a timer at 7:30 am for breakfast, 10:30 am for your morning snack, 1:30 pm for lunch, 4:30 pm for your afternoon snack, 7:30 pm for dinner, and 10:30 pm for evening snack (if necessary).

Take note that you will need to distribute your ideal daily recommended number of calories among your meals so that you are sure to hit your health goals.

Step 3: Decide on how you should prepare your meals.

Your meal plan should be more than just a list of the food you need to eat per mealtime; it should also be your guide in preparing your food. More often than not, you would not have the luxury of time to prepare elaborate meals during busy work days so the next best strategy is to make your meals ahead of time. Doing so will keep you stress-free and on track with regard to your keto diet. Of course, if you do have the time and energy to cook before each mealtime then this is an ideal setup.

To prepare your meals ahead of time, you will need to choose a specific time of the week for buying all of your ingredients in bulk and another time for cooking them all and storing them appropriately in the freezer or refrigerator. Usually, this takes place on a Sunday afternoon.

The first thing you need to do is choose recipes for your meals. A highly practical guide for super busy individuals would be as three sets of recipes: one for Monday, Wednesday, and Friday, one for Tuesday, Saturday, and one for Thursday and Sunday.

Here is an example of three sets of meal plans following the Standard Keto Diet and using the recipes in the succeeding chapters:

Set 1 for Monday, Wednesday and Friday (to be stored in separate containers in the refrigerator except for the smoothies)

Breakfast and Morning Snack: Keto Espresso Smoothie, Coconut Banana Raisin Pancakes (3 servings)
Lunch and Afternoon Snack: Baked Cheesy Chicken Balls, Grilled Radicchio with Balsamic Vinaigrette (3 servings)
Dinner and Evening Snack: Poblano Peppers Stuffed with Pork and Cheese, Buttered Spinach with Shallots and Bacon (3 servings)

Set 2 for Tuesday and Saturday (to be stored in separate containers in the freezer)

Breakfast and Morning Snack: Avocado and Raspberry Smoothie, Cheddar Flapjacks (2 servings)

Lunch and Afternoon Snack: Tex Mex Turkey Salad, Cheesy Broccoli (2 servings)

Dinner and Evening Snack: Stewed Beef and Mushrooms, Avocado and Cucumber Salad (2 servings)

Set 3 for Thursday and Sunday (to be stored in separate containers in the freezer)

Breakfast and Morning Snack: Coconut Spice Smoothie, Bacon Avocado Breakfast Muffins (2 servings)

Lunch and Afternoon Snack: Chicken Barbecue Stew, Cheddar Broccoli Biscuits (2 servings)

Dinner and Evening Snack: Cheesy Tuna and Cauliflower Casserole, Savory Roasted Spaghetti Squash with Kale (2 servings)

With a meal plan system such as this, all you will need to do for the rest of the week is reheat and serve. Continue to adjust your meal plan based on your personal schedule, the types of food you want to eat while on the keto diet, and whatever is available on the market. Make it a habit to prepare your own keto meals and keep things simple and streamlined so that meal planning becomes a sustainable part of your lifestyle.

Chapter 4 – Breakfast Recipes

Get your metabolism revved up at the start of the day by enjoying a healthy, delicious ketogenic breakfast meal. Keto breakfast dishes are high in healthy fats, fiber, lean protein and lots of nutrients from herbs and other fresh ingredients. Serve yours with a hot cup of black coffee or tea, or even just a tall, cold glass of lemon water.

Adding just a bit of sliced fruit on the side won't hurt either.

The following keto breakfast recipes can be prepared during the previous night and then refrigerated to be reheated and served for breakfast the following day. Of course, fresh is always best so find the time to wake up just a bit earlier to prepare breakfast for it is truly worth the effort.

Breakfast Meals

Herb and Mushroom Egg Scramble
Makes 4 servings

Ingredients:
- 1 Tbsp olive oil
- 4 large organic eggs
- 2 cups sliced fresh mushrooms
- 1 small onion, minced
- 5 oz grated cheddar cheese
- 2 Tbsp chopped fresh or 2 tsp dried flat leaf parsley

- 2 Tbsp chopped fresh or 2 tsp dried dill
- ½ Tbsp chopped fresh or ½ tsp dried thyme
- Sea salt
- Freshly ground black pepper

Procedure:
Beat the eggs and season with salt and pepper. Set aside
Place a cast iron skillet over medium high flame and heat through. Once hot, add half the olive oil and reduce to medium flame.

Add the onion and mushroom, then sauté until tender. Stir in the herbs and sauté for 1 minute or until fragrant and wilted, if using fresh. Transfer to a plate and set aside.
Wipe the skillet to clean it. Heat what's left of remaining olive oil. Then add the beaten eggs and scramble until halfway done.

Return the mushroom and herb mixture into the skillet and mix well with the scrambled egg. Cook until the egg is done to a desired consistency.

Transfer to a plate and serve right away.

Coconut Banana Raisin Pancakes
Makes 3 servings

Ingredients:
- 3 large organic eggs
- ¼ cup coconut flour
- 1 Tbsp coconut milk
- 1 Tbsp ground cinnamon
- ¼ tsp ground nutmeg
- ¼ tsp baking soda
- 1 cup raisins
- 2 small ripe bananas, mashed
- Nonstick cooking spray
- Grass-fed butter

Procedure:
Sift the flour, cinnamon, nutmeg, and baking soda in a bowl. Set aside.

Whisk the eggs, mashed banana, and milk together, then mix in the flour mixture until thoroughly incorporated.

Place a pancake griddle over medium high flame and lightly coat with nonstick cooking spray, if needed.

Pour a quarter cup of the batter on the griddle and sprinkle some raisins on top.

Cook for 1 to 2 minutes per side, or until firm. Repeat with the rest of the batter.

Best served warm with butter.

Cheddar Flapjacks
Makes 4 servings

Ingredients:
- 2 Tbsp olive oil
- 2 large egg whites
- ¼ cup water
- 1 cup almond flour
- ½ tsp baking powder
- 2 oz grated cheddar cheese
- 1 garlic clove, minced
- ½ Tbsp chopped green onion
- Grass-fed butter
- Nonstick cooking spray

Procedure:
Whisk the egg whites and water until thoroughly combined. Then, fold in the cheese, almond flour, baking powder, garlic, and green onion.

Gradually pour in the olive oil as you mix until the batter is well incorporated.

Place a pancake griddle over medium high flame and lightly coat with nonstick cooking spray, if needed.

Pour a quarter cup of the batter on the griddle and cook for 1 to 2 minutes per side, or until firm. Repeat with the rest of the batter.

Best served warm with butter.

Bacon Avocado Breakfast Muffins
Makes 24 servings

Ingredients:

- 8 large organic eggs
- 3 Tbsp freshly squeezed lemon juice
- 4 avocados, pitted and peeled
- 3 cups coconut milk
- 10 slices unprocessed bacon
- 1 cup almond flour
- ½ cup ground flaxseeds
- 3 Tbsp ground psyllium husks
- 9 oz Colby Jack cheese
- 2 tsp minced garlic
- 2 tsp dried cilantro
- 2 tsp dried chives
- ½ tsp red chili flakes
- 2 tsp baking powder
- 6 spring onions, minced
- Sea salt
- Freshly ground black pepper

Procedure:
Set the oven to 350 degrees F. Lightly grease 24 muffin tins with butter and set aside.

Place a cast iron skillet over medium high flame and heat through. Add the bacon and cook until crisp. Transfer to a plate lined with paper towels and set aside.

Combine the almond flour with the ground flaxseeds, psyllium husks, dried spices, baking powder and chili flakes.

Combine the avocado with the eggs, lemon juice and coconut milk. Mash well until thoroughly incorporated.

Combine the almond flour mixture with the avocado mixture until well incorporated. Fold in the cheese, garlic, and green onion. Season to taste with salt and pepper.

Divide the mixture among the muffin tins, then bake for 25 minutes, or until muffins are firm and golden brown.

Serve warm. Muffins can be stored in the freezer for up to 3 weeks and reheated in the broiler before serving.

Bacon Ricotta Breakfast Muffins
Makes 24 servings

Ingredients:
- 10 slices unprocessed bacon
- 2 cups grated Parmesan cheese
- 2 lb ricotta cheese
- 20 oz baby spinach, washed and drained thoroughly
- 1 cup plain yogurt
- 4 large eggs
- 4 oz chopped pine nuts
- Sea salt

- Freshly ground black pepper
- Grass-fed butter

Procedure:

Set the oven to 350 degrees F. Lightly grease 24 muffin tins with butter and set aside.

Boil salted water in a saucepan, then blanch the baby spinach for 30 seconds. Drain thoroughly, then mince and set aside.

Mince the bacon and place in a bowl. Fold in the spinach, cheeses, yogurt, and eggs. Season with a bit of salt and pepper, then pour the batter into the prepared muffin tins.

Top with pine nuts, then bake for 30 minutes, or until the muffins are firm and tops are golden brown.

Serve warm. Muffins can be stored in the freezer for up to 3 weeks and reheated in the broiler before serving.

Creamy Keto Porridge
Makes 4 servings

Ingredients:

- ½ cup unsweetened shredded coconut
- 2 Tbsp oat bran
- 2 Tbsp ground flaxseeds
- 1 tsp ground cinnamon
- 1 cup heavy cream

- 2 cups water
- Sea salt
- 1 Tbsp grass-fed butter

Procedure:
Combine the shredded coconut, oat bran and flaxseed meal in a saucepan, then stir in the cinnamon, heavy cream, water, and a pinch of salt.

Place over medium low flame and bring to a boil. Once boiling, immediately turn off the heat and stir.

Divide the mixture among four bowls. Let stand for 5 minutes, or until slightly thickened. Add a quarter tablespoon of butter on top of each serving, then serve warm.

Double Cheese Waffles
Makes 6 servings

Ingredients:
- 1 ½ cups chopped cauliflower florets
- 1 cup grated mozzarella cheese
- ¼ cup grated Parmesan cheese
- 2 large organic eggs
- 1 Tbsp chopped fresh chives
- 1 tsp onion powder
- 1 tsp garlic powder
- ½ tsp freshly ground black pepper
- Sea salt

- Grass-fed butter

Procedure:
Place the cauliflower florets in a food processor and pulse until crumbly. Transfer to a mixing bowl.

Fold the cheeses, eggs, chives, onion and garlic powders, black pepper, and a pinch of salt into the crumbled cauliflower. Mix very well.

Prepare the waffle maker based on manufacturer's instructions.

Pour just enough of the batter to fill the waffle maker, then cook for approximately 5 minutes or more.

Transfer to a plate and serve with butter.

Waffles can be made the previous night; simply refrigerate and reheat in the waffle maker the next morning.

Breakfast Smoothies

Keto Espresso Smoothie
Makes 2 servings

Ingredients:
- 2 scoops protein powder, no carbs
- 2 espresso shots
- ½ cup full fat Greek yogurt
- 2 cups ice cubes
- Cinnamon
- Liquid stevia

Procedure:
Pour the espresso, yogurt, protein powder, and ice cubes into a high power blender. Cover the blender, and then blend on high until smooth.

Add cinnamon and liquid stevia to taste, and then blend again. Pour into a tall glass and consume right away.

Avocado and Raspberry Smoothie
Makes 1 serving

Ingredients:
- ½ cup vanilla almond milk
- ½ cup diced avocado
- ½ Tbsp heavy cream
- ½ scoop protein powder, no carb
- 2 Tbsp frozen raspberries
- Liquid stevia

Procedure:
Combine the almond milk, avocado, heavy cream, and protein powder in a high power blender. Cover the blender, then blend on high until smooth.

Add the frozen raspberries and pulse until smooth with bits of raspberries still intact. Sweeten to taste with liquid stevia and blend again.

Pour into a tall glass and consume right away.

Green Blueberry Yogurt Smoothie
Makes 2 servings

Ingredients:
- 4 cups baby spinach leaves
- 1 cup full fat Greek yogurt
- 1 cup frozen blueberries
- 2 cups ice cubes
- 3 Tbsp coconut oil
- 2 Tbsp chia seeds

Procedure:
Pour the yogurt, ice cubes, coconut oil, chia seeds, and spinach leaves into a high power blender. Cover the blender, then blend on high until smooth.

Add the blueberries and pulse until smooth, with bits of blueberries still intact. Pour into a tall glass and consume right away.

Coconut Spice Smoothie
Makes 1 serving

Ingredients:
- ½ cup coconut milk
- 2 Tbsp unsweetened shredded coconut
- 1 Tbsp almond butter
- ½ Tbsp ground flaxseeds
- ½ Tbsp pure vanilla extract
- ½ tsp ground cinnamon
- ½ tsp ground ginger
- 3 ice cubes

Procedure:
Pour the coconut milk, almond butter, ground flaxseeds, vanilla extract, spices, and ice cubes in the blender.

Cover the blender, then blend on high until smooth. Pour into a tall glass and consume right away.

Spiced Sweet Potato Smoothie
Makes 2 servings

Ingredients:
- 2 small sweet potatoes, peeled, boiled, and cubed
- 1 ½ cups vanilla almond milk
- ¼ cup avocado
- 2 scoops protein powder, no carb
- 2 tsp pure vanilla extract
- 1 tsp ground cinnamon
- ½ tsp ground nutmeg
- ½ tsp ground allspice

Procedure:
Place the sweet potato into the blender, then add the almond milk, avocado, protein powder, vanilla extract, and spices.

Cover the blender, then blend on high until smooth. Pour into a tall glass and consume right away.

Peanut Butter Smoothie
Makes 1 serving

Ingredients:
- ½ cup vanilla almond milk
- ½ cup ice cubes
- ¼ cup coconut milk
- 1 Tbsp smooth peanut butter, natural
- ½ tsp pure vanilla extract
- Liquid stevia

Procedure:
Pour the almond milk, coconut milk, ice cubes, vanilla extract, and peanut butter in a high power blender.
Cover the blender, then blend on high until smooth. Sweeten to taste with liquid stevia, then blend again to combine.

Pour into a tall glass and consume right away.

Buttered Pumpkin Spice Latte
Makes 2 servings

Ingredients:
- 1 cup brewed coffee
- 4 Tbsp pureed pumpkin
- 2 Tbsp almond milk
- 2 Tbsp grass-fed butter
- ½ tsp pumpkin pie spice
- Liquid stevia

Procedure:
Combine the almond milk, brewed coffee, butter, pureed pumpkin, and pumpkin pie spice in a high power blender. Cover the blender, then blend on high until smooth.

Sweeten to taste with liquid stevia and blend again. Pour into a tall glass and consume right away.

Chapter 5 – Lunch Recipes

Keto lunch dishes are highly satisfying and full of energy and nutrients from fresh ingredients. Choose only the best organic ingredients from your local farmer's market and do not hesitate to opt for fresher, locally produced alternatives instead of the usual ingredients listed. The key to a healthy keto diet is in the quality of the produce, after all.

Follow any of these healthy keto lunch recipes to prepare lunch meals ahead of time. Store the meals in airtight lunch boxes and refrigerate. That way, all you will have to do later on is reheat in the microwave or enjoy chilled. It helps to pack a thermos full of hot green tea to not only make your lunch more special, but also to help boost your metabolism and maximize your body's fat-burning power.

Main Course Recipes

Baked Cheesy Chicken Balls
Makes 12 servings

Ingredients:
- ½ lb ground chicken breast
- ½ cup almond flour
- ½ cup tomato sauce

- ¼ cup grated Parmesan cheese
- 1.5 oz fresh mozzarella cheese
- ¼ cup full cream milk
- ½ tsp sea salt
- ¼ tsp dried oregano
- Freshly ground black pepper
- Nonstick cooking spray

Procedure:
Set the oven to 350 degrees F. Lightly coat a baking dish with nonstick cooking spray and set aside.

Combine the parmesan, milk, salt, oregano, and half the almond flour in a bowl. Mix well, and then fold in the ground chicken. Mix until well incorporated.

Divide the mixture into 12 equal sized balls and dredge each in the remaining flour.

Arrange the chicken balls on the prepared baking dish, and then bake for 20 minutes, turning the balls once halfway through the cooking time.

Pour the tomato sauce over the baked chicken balls, and then add the mozzarella cheese on top.

Bake again for 12 minutes, or until the mozzarella is melted. Best served warm with a fresh green salad.

Greek Tuna Salad
Makes 6 servings

Ingredients:

- 15 oz BPA-free canned white albacore tuna in oil, drained
- ¾ cup extra virgin olive oil
- 1 ½ cups crumbled feta cheese
- 1/3 cup chopped green olives
- 1/3 cup chopped fresh flat leaf parsley
- ¾ cup diced roasted red bell peppers
- 1 ½ Tbsp freshly squeezed lemon juice
- 1 ½ Tbsp chopped capers
- 3 cups endive leaves
- Sea salt
- Freshly ground black pepper

Procedure:
Arrange the endive leaves on a serving plate and set aside. Crumble the tuna with clean hands, then mix in the olive oil, feta cheese, green olives, lemon juice, capers, parsley, and roasted red bell peppers. Mix well.

Season to taste with salt and pepper, then spoon the mixture on top of the bed of endive leaves. Serve right away.

Chicken Barbecue Stew
Makes 4 servings

Ingredients:
- 2 Tbsp olive oil
- 4 chicken thighs
- 2 cups chicken stock, low sodium
- 2 cups beef stock, low sodium
- 3 tsp chili powder
- Sea salt
- Freshly ground black pepper

For the Barbecue Sauce:
- 1/3 cup tomato sauce
- 1/3 cup tomato paste
- 3 Tbsp Dijon mustard
- 1 ½ tsp low sodium soy sauce
- 1 ½ Tbsp Tabasco sauce
- 3 tsp liquid smoke
- 1 ½ tsp Worcestershire sauce
- 2 tsp garlic powder
- 1 ½ tsp chili powder
- 1 ½ tsp garlic powder
- 1 ½ tsp red chili flakes
- 1 ½ tsp cumin
- 1/3 cup grass-fed butter

Procedure:
Mix together all the ingredients for the barbecue sauce, then set aside.

Set the oven to 400 degrees F. Line a baking sheet with aluminum foil and set aside.
Remove the chicken meat from the bones, then season the meat with chili powder.

Lay the chicken meat on the prepared baking sheet and bake for 45 minutes.

Place a stockpot over medium high flame and heat through. Once hot, add the olive oil and swirl to coat.

Sauté the chicken bones for 5 minutes, then stir in the chicken and beef stocks.

Once the chicken meat is cooked, remove the skin and add the roasted chicken meat to the pot. Mix well until combined.

Stir in the barbecue sauce and mix well. Let simmer for 15 minutes, then ladle into soup bowls and serve right away with a fresh green salad.

Avocado Beef Patties

Makes 2 servings

Ingredients:
- ½ lb lean organic ground beef
- 1 small avocado, pitted and peeled
- ¼ Tbsp freshly squeezed lemon juice
- 2 slices yellow cheddar cheese, 1 oz each
- 1 tomato, diced
- 1 small onion, sliced into thin rings
- 4 romaine or iceberg lettuce leaves
- Sea salt
- Freshly ground black pepper

Procedure:
Lay the lettuce leaves on two serving dishes and set aside. Divide the ground beef into two patties. Make compact, then season with salt and pepper.

Prepare the stovetop grill. Grill the beef patties for 5 to 8 minutes per side or until cooked through.

Lay a patty over each bed of lettuce.

Slice the avocado into thin pieces. Sprinkle the lemon juice over the sliced avocado to prevent them from browning.

Lay the sliced avocado on top of the burger patties, then add the chopped garlic and onion rings on top. Serve right away with yellow mustard, if desired.

Oriental Style Chicken Salad
Makes 4 servings

Ingredients:
- 4 cups torn lettuce
- 2 ½ cups shredded cooked chicken
- 4 slices unprocessed bacon
- 1 ½ cups shredded cabbage
- 3 Tbsp diced canned water chestnuts
- 3 Tbsp shredded carrot
- 5 green onions, chopped
- 1/3 cup slivered almonds
- 1 ½ Tbsp sesame seeds
- ¾ Tbsp grass-fed butter

For the Sesame Dressing:
- 3 Tbsp low sodium soy sauce
- 2 Tbsp rice vinegar
- 1 Tbsp dark sesame oil
- 1 garlic clove, crushed
- 2 tsp freshly squeezed lemon juice
- 1/3 tsp freshly ground black pepper

Procedure:
Combine all the ingredients for the dressing in a bowl, then set aside.

Combine the lettuce, cabbage, carrot, chestnuts, and green onion. Refrigerate until ready to serve.

Place a cast iron skillet over medium high flame and cook the bacon to a crisp. Set aside on a plate lined with paper towels.

In the same skillet, cook the almonds, sesame seeds, and butter until golden brown. Transfer to a plate.

Take the vegetables out of the refrigerator, then add the dressing and almond and sesame seed mixture. Toss well to combine.

Divide among four plates and add the chicken on top, followed by the bacon. Serve chilled or warm.

Pork and Mushroom Meatballs

Makes 2 servings

Ingredients:
- ¾ lb organic lean ground pork
- ½ cup minced fresh mushrooms, any kind
- ½ Tbsp low sodium soy sauce
- 1 Tbsp chopped green onion
- ¼ tsp sesame oil
- 1 small organic egg
- 1/8 tsp garlic powder
- ¼ tsp sea salt
- 1/8 tsp freshly ground black pepper

Procedure:
Place the ground pork in a bowl, and then fold in the minced mushrooms. Add the soy sauce, salt, pepper, garlic powder, green onion, egg, and sesame oil.

Mix well, and then form into small inch sized balls.

Boil water in a saucepan over medium high flame, and then add the meatballs. Cover and simmer over medium flame for about 10 minutes, or until the meatballs are completely cooked.

Transfer the meatballs to a bowl using a slotted spoon then serve warm, preferably with a green salad.

Tex Mex Turkey Salad
Makes 2 servings

Ingredients:
- 1 cup cooked diced turkey
- 2 cups chopped cauliflower florets
- 1 small red bell pepper, seeded and diced
- 1 small red onion, diced
- 2 Tbsp chopped canned green chilies
- 3 oz Monterey Jack cheese, cubed
- 2 Tbsp chopped black olives
- 3 Tbsp mayonnaise
- ½ Tbsp white wine vinegar
- ¾ tsp freshly squeezed lime juice
- ½ tsp chili powder
- ¼ tsp ground cumin
- ¼ tsp dried oregano
- 2 Tbsp chopped fresh cilantro

Procedure:
Combine the mayonnaise, oregano, chili powder, cumin, vinegar, and lime juice in a bowl. Refrigerate until ready to serve.

Steam the cauliflower florets in a bowl of water in the microwave or in a steamer basket over boiling water for 5 minutes, or until tender.

Drain the cauliflower, then transfer to a bowl and allow to cool slightly. Add the bell pepper, red onion, green chilies, black olives, cooked diced turkey, and cubed cheese. Toss well to combine.

Add the dressing and fold gently to coat. Garnish with fresh cilantro, then serve.

Side Dish or Snack Recipes

Grilled Radicchio with Balsamic Vinaigrette
Makes 9 servings

Ingredients:
- 2 radicchios, sliced into thin wedges
- 1 ½ Tbsp balsamic vinegar
- 1 ½ Tbsp extra virgin olive oil
- Sea salt

Procedure:
Set the broiler to high heat.

Whisk together the balsamic vinegar, olive oil, and a pinch of sea salt. Mix well, then add the radicchio wedges and toss well to coat.

Spread the radicchio wedges on the broiler pan, then broil for 5 minutes per side, or until grilled tightly.

Set on a cooling rack and allow to cool slightly, then store in a glass bowl. Cover and serve right away, or refrigerate.

Cheesy Broccoli
Makes 6 servings

Ingredients:
- 3 cups chopped broccoli florets
- ¾ cup shredded sharp Cheddar cheese
- 1/3 cup heavy cream
- 1/3 Tbsp ranch dressing
- Sea salt
- Freshly ground black pepper

Procedure:
Set the oven to 375 degrees F.

Combine the ranch dressing, cheddar cheese, and heavy cream. Season to taste with salt and pepper, and then add the chopped broccoli. Mix well until combined.

Pour the mixture into the casserole dish, and then spread out. Bake for 20 to 30 minutes, or until the cheese is bubbly and the broccoli is fork tender.

Best served warm.

Cheddar Broccoli Biscuits
Makes 6 to 8 servings

Ingredients:
- ½ cup melted coconut oil, cooled
- 3 cups almond flour
- 8 cups chopped broccoli florets
- 4 large organic eggs
- 1 tsp apple cider vinegar
- 1 tsp baking soda
- 2 tsp garlic powder
- 2 tsp paprika
- 2 tsp sea salt
- 2 tsp freshly ground black pepper

Procedure:
Set the oven to 375 degrees F. Line a baking sheet with parchment paper and set aside.

Place the broccoli in a food processor and process until minced. Work in batches.

Combine the almond flour and spices in a mixing bowl, and then mix in the coconut oil, vinegar, and eggs. Mix well to form a dough.

Fold in the broccoli and Cheddar cheese, mixing well.

Divide the mixture into 24 balls, and then press the balls on the prepared baking sheet, leaving over an inch of space between each piece.

Bake for 5 minutes, then set on a cooling rack and allow to cool slightly. Serve right away or store in an airtight container.

Mashed Cauliflower and Turnip
Makes 4 servings

Ingredients:
- ½ lb chopped cauliflower
- ½ lb fresh turnips
- ¼ cup heavy cream
- ¼ cup grass-fed butter
- Sea salt

Procedure:
Place the turnips and cauliflower in a pot, then add enough water to cover them by an about two inches. Add a generous pinch of salt.

Place over high flame and bring to a boil. Boil for 12 minutes or until extra tender. Drain thoroughly, then return to the pot and add the heavy cream and butter.

Mash everything until smooth, then serve right away or transfer to an airtight container and refrigerate.

Baked Garlic Parmesan Cauliflower
Makes 3 servings

Ingredients:
- 3 cups chopped cauliflower florets
- 4 Tbsp grass-fed butter
- 3 Tbsp shredded Parmesan cheese
- 2 garlic cloves, minced
- Sea salt

Procedure:
Set the oven to 350 degrees F.

Combine the butter and garlic in a saucepan, then place over low flame. Heat until the garlic is golden. Set aside.

Spread the cauliflower on a rimmed baking sheet, then pour the garlic butter on top and add salt and Parmesan cheese.

Bake for 15 minutes, or until the cauliflower is crisp tender. Serve right away.

Basic Cauliflower Rice
Makes 4 servings

Ingredients:
- 1 small cauliflower head
- 3 Tbsp water
- Sea salt
- Freshly ground black pepper

Procedure:
Rinse the cauliflower thoroughly, then chop and place in a food processor. Process until grainy, similar to rice grains.

Transfer the cauliflower rice to a microwaveable bowl, then add a pinch of salt and pepper. Add the water, then microwave for 2 minutes or until tender, but still firm.

Adjust seasoning to taste, if needed, then serve or store in an airtight container.

Tomato, Olive and Mozzarella Salad
Makes 2 servings

Ingredients:
- 1 ½ cups cherry tomatoes, halved
- 1 ½ cups pitted kalamata olives
- 1 ½ cups torn mozzarella cheese

Procedure:
In a bowl, combine the tomatoes, olives, and mozzarella cheese.

Serve right away, or store in an airtight container and refrigerate until ready to serve.

Chapter 6 – Dinner Recipes

inner should be treated as a special occasion every night and not just to celebrate a certain event. When you take the time to savor and appreciate the flavors of your meals, you become more likely to choose healthy food. A simple change of ambiance such as lit candles and music in tune with the theme of your dinner will make a big difference.

Follow these keto dinner recipes to present delicious and nutrient-packed dishes that are sure to make you look forward to your evening meals all the time. You can even serve with a hot cup of herbal tea to make it all the more relaxing. And, just like the lunch recipes, these dinner recipes call for organic and fresh ingredients. Choose the highest quality that your budget can afford because sure enough, your body deserves only the best.

Main Course Recipes

Poblano Peppers Stuffed with Pork and Cheese
Makes 3 to 4 servings

Ingredients:
- ¾ cup olive oil
- 1 ½ lb organic lean ground pork
- 2 cups freshly grated cheddar cheese
- 4 large poblano peppers

- 1 ½ cups salsa, unsweetened
- 1 ½ tsp chili powder
- 1 ½ Tbsp ground flaxseeds

Procedure:
Set the oven to 425 degrees F.

Halve the peppers lengthwise, then scoop out the seeds. Rinse the peppers and set aside to drain on paper towels.

Place a cast iron skillet over high flame and heat through. Add the olive oil, then sauté the ground pork with the chili powder until pork is crumbly and browned.

Remove from heat and fold in 1 ½ cups of cheddar cheese. Mix well until the cheese is melted.

Pour the salsa into a baking dish.

Stuff the halved peppers with the pork and cheese mixture, then arrange them on the prepared baking dish, cut sides facing up.

Top the stuffed peppers with the remaining cheddar cheese.

Bake the stuffed peppers for 30 minutes, uncovered. Sprinkle the ground flaxseed on top, then serve warm.

Sea Bass and Spinach with Coconut Lemon Sauce
Makes 2 servings

Ingredients:
- 2 large sea bass fillets (or salmon or halibut)
- 4 cups fresh spinach
- ½ cup coconut milk
- 2 ½ Tbsp freshly squeezed lemon juice
- 2 Tbsp pine nuts
- 2 Tbsp chopped fresh flat leaf parsley
- 2 Tbsp grass-fed butter
- Sea salt

Procedure:
Season the fish fillets on both sides with sea salt, then set aside.

Rinse and drain the spinach thoroughly, then dry in a colander or salad spinner. Set aside.

Place a cast iron skillet over medium high flame and heat through. Add half the butter in the skillet and reduce to medium flame. Cook the fillets for 4 minutes per side or until golden brown.

In the meantime, place another skillet over medium flame and heat the remaining butter. Sauté the spinach until wilted, then stir in the pine nuts and sauté until lightly toasted.

Place a saucepan over low flame and add the coconut milk. Stir in the parsley and lemon juice. Cook until heated through; do not boil.

Spread the spinach on the serving plate, then add the fish fillets on top. Spoon the sauce over the fillets, then serve right away.

Stewed Beef and Mushrooms
Makes 2 servings

Ingredients:
- ¼ cup olive oil
- 25 grams grass-fed butter
- ½ lb cubed stew beef
- ½ quart bone or beef broth
- ½ lb sliced fresh mushrooms, any kind
- ¼ cup diced onion
- ½ Tbsp ground flaxseeds
- ½ tsp minced garlic
- ½ tsp dried thyme
- 1 bay leaf
- 2 Tbsp chopped fresh parsley
- Sea salt
- Freshly ground black pepper
-

Procedure:
Place a stock pot over medium high flame and heat through. Add the olive oil and butter, then stir in the cubed beef. Cook until browned all over.

Stir in the onion and mushrooms, then sauté until tender. Stir in the garlic, bay leaf, thyme, and ground flaxseeds, then stir in the broth.

Bring to a boil, then reduce to low flame and simmer for 1 hour or until the beef is extra tender.

Discard the bay leaf. If desired, remove the cubed beef and shred using two forks. Stir back into the stew followed by the parsley.

Ladle into soup bowls and serve piping hot.

Cheesy Tuna and Cauliflower Casserole
Makes 9 servings

Ingredients:
- 18 oz canned chunky tuna
- ¾ cup chopped celery
- 1 ½ large cauliflower heads
- ½ cup chopped green onion
- 3 small zucchini, scrubbed and sliced
- 3 cups shredded cheddar or Monterey Jack cheese
- 2 small tomatoes, chopped
- 1 cup sour cream
- ¾ cup mayonnaise
- 3 tsp yellow mustard
- ¾ tsp dried thyme
- Sea salt
- Freshly ground black pepper

Procedure:
Set the oven to 350 degrees F.

Drain the tuna, then crumble in a bowl and fold in the green onion and celery.

Chop the cauliflower, then place in a steamer basket and steam over a pot of boiling water for 5 minutes or until fork tender.

Combine the tuna with the steamed cauliflower and mix well.

In a separate bowl, combine the mayonnaise, sour cream, thyme, mustard, salt, and pepper. Pour the mixture over the tuna and cauliflower mixture, then combine everything well.

Pack the mixture into a casserole dish, then lay the sliced zucchini on top. Sprinkle the cheese on top, then bake for 40 minutes, or until the casserole is bubbly hot.

Top with chopped tomato, then serve warm.

Crusted Fish Fillets with Dilled Sauce
Makes 4 servings

Ingredients:
- 1 ½ lb white fish fillets, wild-caught
- 1 large organic egg
- 1 cup freshly grated Parmesan cheese
- 1/3 tsp chili powder
- ¾ tsp dried parsley
- 1 cup almond meal
- 3 Tbsp organic mayonnaise
- 1/3 tsp sea salt
- Freshly ground black pepper
- Coconut oil

For the Dilled Sauce:
- 2/3 cup organic mayonnaise
- 2/3 cup sour cream
- 3 Tbsp chopped fresh dill
- 2 Tbsp chopped capers, drained
- 3 tsp freshly squeezed lemon juice
- Optional: 3 dill pickles, diced

Procedure:
Combine all the ingredients for the dilled sauce in a bowl, then cover and refrigerate until ready to serve.

In a shallow bowl, combine the Parmesan cheese, almond meal, chili powder, dried parsley, salt, and a pinch of black pepper. Mix well.

Beat the egg in a bowl, then stir in the mayo.

Slice the fish fillets into 1 inch by 2 inch strips. Coat in the egg mixture, then dredge in the cheese and almond meal mixture. Set aside.

Place a cast iron skillet over medium high flame and add about a half inch of coconut oil. Reduce to medium flame and heat through, then add the fish and cook for 2 minutes per side, or until golden brown and completely cooked.

Drain on a plate lined with paper towels, then arrange on a serving dish. Spoon the sauce into a dipping bowl, then serve.

Beef Chili
Makes 3 servings

Ingredients:
* 1 lb lean organic ground beef
* 1 quart bone or beef stock, low sodium
* ¼ cup olive oil
* 2 Tbsp ground flaxseeds
* 1/3 cup minced yellow onion
* 1 Tbsp chili powder
* 1 tsp dried oregano
* ½ tsp ground cumin
* ¼ tsp garlic powder
* Sea salt
* Freshly ground black pepper

Procedure:
Place a stockpot over high flame and heat through. Stir in the ground beef, then add the chili powder, cumin, garlic powder, and onion.

Sauté until the beef is browned and crumbly, then stir in the olive oil, beef broth, and ground flaxseeds. Bring the mixture to a boil.

Once boiling, reduce to a simmer over medium high flame. Simmer, uncovered, for about 30 minutes to an hour or until the chili is thickened.

Season to taste with salt and pepper and serve piping hot. If desired, store the beef chili in the refrigerator and reheat the following day.

Caribbean Chicken Stew
Makes 4 servings

Ingredients:
- 2 ½ lb chopped chicken pieces
- ½ quart chicken stock, low sodium
- 1 carrot, peeled and sliced
- ¾ cup cubed pumpkin
- ¾ cup cubed rutabaga
- ½ small turnip, cubed
- ½ cup chopped cauliflower florets
- 1 ½ cups shredded cabbage
- ½ tsp Tabasco sauce

For the marinade:
- 2 Tbsp freshly squeezed lime juice
- ¾ cup diced celery
- 1 small onion, minced
- 1 small ripe green bell pepper, seeded and chopped
- ½ Tbsp ground cumin
- ¼ tsp chicken bouillon granules
- ¼ tsp ground nutmeg

Procedure:
Combine all the ingredients for the marinade in a food processor and blend until smooth. Pour into a large bowl and add the chicken pieces. Turn several times to coat.

Cover the bowl and refrigerate to marinate the chicken for 8 hours, or overnight.

To cook, pour the chicken stock into the pot with the chicken pieces and marinade. Place over high flame and bring to a boil.

Once boiling, reduce to a simmer over low flame. Cover and simmer for 45 minutes to an hour, or until the chicken is cooked through.

Remove the chicken pieces from the pot and transfer to a plate. Strain the broth and discard any solids.

Pour the strained broth back into the pot and place over medium flame. Add the pumpkin, turnip, rutabaga and carrot, then simmer for 20 minutes.

Meanwhile, remove the bones from the chicken pieces, then stir into the pot. Mix everything well, then add the cauliflower and cabbage. Simmer for 20 minutes, then serve.

Side Dish Recipes

Buttered Spinach with Shallots and Bacon
Makes 3 servings

Ingredients:
- 8 oz spinach
- ¼ lb unprocessed bacon
- ¼ cup chopped shallots
- ¼ cup chopped white onion
- 1 Tbsp grass-fed butter

Procedure:
Dice the bacon and set aside.

Place a cast iron skillet over medium high flame and heat through. Once hot, add the bacon and sauté the bacon with the shallots and onion. Sauté for 12 minutes or until the onion is caramelized.

Reduce to medium flame, then stir in the spinach and sauté to combine. Cover the skillet and cook for 3 minutes or until the spinach is wilted.

Transfer to a serving plate, then serve right away.

Avocado and Cucumber Salad
Makes 4 servings

Ingredients:
- 1 cup diced English cucumber
- ½ cup diced avocado
- 1 small onion, diced
- 1 Tbsp freshly squeezed lime juice
- 1 Tbsp extra virgin olive oil
- Garlic powder
- Red pepper flakes
- Sea salt
- Freshly ground black pepper

Procedure:
Place the avocado in a bowl, then add the lime juice and toss gently to coat. Add the cucumber, onion, and olive oil, then toss again to coat.

Season to taste with salt, pepper, garlic powder, and red pepper flakes. Toss well, then cover and refrigerate until ready to serve.

Savory Roasted Spaghetti Squash with Kale
Makes 3 servings

Ingredients:
- Olive oil
- ½ spaghetti squash
- 2 cups chopped kale leaves
- 1 small onion, minced
- ½ tsp balsamic vinegar
- ¼ tsp chili powder
- Sea salt
- Freshly ground black pepper

Procedure:
Set the oven to 350 degrees F.

Scoop out the seeds and pulp from the spaghetti squash, then place it, exposed side facing upward, on the baking sheet. Brush with olive oil.

Bake the squash for 45 minutes to 1 hour, or until the squash is extra tender.

Meanwhile, place a skillet over medium high flame and heat through. Add half a tablespoon of olive oil, then sauté the onion until tender.

Stir in the kale and season with salt and pepper. Sauté until the kale is almost wilted and the onions are tender. Transfer to a plate and set aside.

Carefully remove the squash from the oven, then scrape out the roasted squash flesh using a fork. Transfer to a bowl.

Drizzle the balsamic vinegar and half a tablespoon of olive oil over the squash, then season to taste with chili powder, salt, and pepper.

Spread out the squash on a serving plate, then top with the kale and serve right away.

Buttered Mushrooms
Makes 3 servings

Ingredients:
- ½ lb fresh mushrooms (such as Portobello)
- 1 Tbsp grass-fed butter
- ½ tsp soy sauce, low sodium

Procedure:
Rinse the mushrooms, then set aside to drain.

Place a cast iron skillet over medium high flame and heat through. Once hot, add the butter, mushrooms, and soy sauce. Sauté until the mushrooms are tender and cooked through.

Transfer to a serving plate, then serve right away.

Mashed Zesty Garlic Cauliflower
Makes 2 servings

Ingredients:
- 2 cups chopped cauliflower florets
- 2 ½ Tbsp mayonnaise
- 1 small garlic clove, peeled
- ½ Tbsp water
- ½ Tbsp chopped fresh chives
- ¼ tsp freshly grated lime or lemon zest
- ¼ tsp sea salt
- Freshly ground black pepper

Procedure:
Combine the garlic, mayonnaise, and sea salt in a microwaveable bowl. Stir in the pinch of black pepper, then set aside.

Add the cauliflower and mix well to combine. Pour in the water, then microwave for 10 minutes, or until the cauliflower is extra tender.

Remove the cauliflower from the microwave and allow to cool completely. Once cooled, transfer to a food processor and add the chives, lemon juice, and zest. Blend until mashed.

Transfer to a serving bowl, then serve right away.

Cheesy Creamed Spinach
Makes 6 servings

Ingredients:
- 15 oz frozen spinach, thawed
- ¾ cup heavy cream
- 1/3 cup Parmesan cheese
- 3 Tbsp grass-fed butter
- Sea salt
- Freshly ground black pepper
- Ground nutmeg

Procedure:
Steam the spinach with a few tablespoons of water in the microwave until wilted. Drain thoroughly, then set aside.

In a saucepan, combine the spinach with the heavy cream, Parmesan cheese, and butter. Simmer over medium flame until cheese is melted. Stir well.

Season to taste with salt, pepper, and nutmeg, then transfer to a serving bowl. Serve right away.

Roasted Asparagus Wrapped in Bacon
Makes 6 servings

Ingredients:
- 2 Tbsp olive oil
- 1 lb asparagus, trimmed
- 6 slices unprocessed bacon
- 2 tsp minced garlic
- 1/3 cup mayonnaise
- 3 tsp freshly squeezed lemon juice
- Red chili flakes
- Sea salt
- Freshly ground black pepper

Procedure:
Set the oven to 400 degrees F. Line a baking sheet with aluminum foil, then set aside.

Divide the asparagus into 6 equal bundles. Wrap a slice of bacon around each bundle, then arrange on the prepared baking sheet.

Drizzle the olive oil over the asparagus bundle, then season with salt, pepper, and red chili flakes.

Bake for 25 minutes, or until the bacon is crisp and cooked through and the asparagus is browned and tender.

Meanwhile, combine the mayonnaise, garlic, lemon juice, and sea salt. Mix well.

Serve the asparagus with the dipping sauce.

Chapter 7 – One Week Meal Plan

The following one week keto meal plan is ideal for those who plan on preparing their meals every day. However, you can also plan on making your meals ahead of time and storing them in the refrigerator for easy reheating later on during the week. The 28 recipes in the previous chapters can be used to make several weeks' worth of meal plans and all you have to do is decide which ones to prep for each day.

Day 1
Breakfast: Herb and Mushroom Egg Scramble and/or Keto Espresso Smoothie
Lunch: (Main Dish) Baked Cheesy Chicken Balls, (Side Dish) Grilled Radicchio with Balsamic Vinaigrette
Dinner: (Main Dish) Poblano Peppers Stuffed with Pork and Cheese, (Side Dish) Buttered Spinach with Shallots and Bacon

Day 2
Breakfast: Coconut Banana Raisin Pancakes and/or Avocado and Raspberry Smoothie
Lunch: (Main Dish) Greek Tuna Salad, (Snack) Cheesy Broccoli
Dinner: (Main Dish) Sea Bass and Spinach with Coconut Lemon Sauce, (Side Dish) Avocado and Cucumber Salad

Day 3

Breakfast: Cheddar Flapjacks and/or Spiced Sweet Potato Smoothie

Lunch: (Main Dish) Chicken Barbecue Stew, (Side Dish) Cheddar Broccoli Biscuits

Dinner: (Main Dish) Stewed Beef and Mushrooms, (Side Dish) Savory Roasted Spaghetti Squash with Kale

Day 4

Breakfast: Bacon Avocado Breakfast Muffins and/or Green Blueberry Yogurt Smoothie

Lunch: (Main Dish) Avocado Beef Patties, (Side Dish) Mashed Cauliflower and Turnip

Dinner: (Main Dish) Cheesy Tuna and Cauliflower Casserole, (Side Dish) Buttered Mushrooms

Day 5

Breakfast: Bacon Ricotta Breakfast Muffins and/or Coconut Spice Smoothie

Lunch: (Main Dish) Oriental Style Chicken Salad, (Snack) Baked Garlic Parmesan Cauliflower

Dinner: (Main Dish) Crusted Fish Fillets with Dilled Sauce, (Side Dish) Mashed Zesty Garlic Cauliflower

Day 6

Breakfast: Creamy Keto Porridge and/or Peanut Butter Smoothie

Lunch: (Main Dish) Pork and Mushroom Meatballs, (Side Dish) Basic Cauliflower Rice

Dinner: (Main Dish) Beef Chili, (Side Dish) Cheesy Creamed Spinach

Day 7

Breakfast: Double Cheese Waffles and/or Buttered Pumpkin Spice Latte

Lunch: (Main Dish) Tex Mex Turkey Salad, (Snack) Tomato, Olive and Mozzarella Salad

Dinner: (Main Dish) Caribbean Chicken Stew, (Side Dish) Roasted Asparagus Wrapped in Bacon

In this one week meal plan, it is also assumed that you will be working out on a regular basis. Doing so will boost your metabolism and trigger your body to burn up your fat stores. On the other hand, if you will not be working out as frequently, then it is advised that you should reduce your portions for each meal from a quarter to half the recommended serving size.

Regardless of whether you are working out or not, you should stay hydrated by drinking lots of water. You should also snack on low carbohydrate vegetables to nourish your body with a variety of vitamins, minerals and other nutrients that it needs.

Conclusion

I hope this book was able to help you to start the keto diet and prepare delicious keto meals efficiently.

The next step is to create sustainable meal plans that will guide you while you are on the keto diet. Continue to stock up on keto foods and find ways to purchase organic ingredients from inexpensive and easily accessible sources. Finally, do not forget to exercise regularly so that you can achieve your health goals effectively.

What to read next

There are millions of books on Amazon. I'm are glad that you discovered my book and got to the end. Thank you for that.

I know the feeling after finishing a good book. The feeling of wanting more.

If you want more, check out my book on weight loss and training, *Intermittent Fasting: Wear Your Favorite Pair of Jeans, Look Good In Photos and Feel Sexy Again!*

Best,
Sebastian Beach

www.ingramcontent.com/pod-product-compliance
Lightning Source LLC
LaVergne TN
LVHW010656200726
843507LV00011B/1892